#FREEDOMCHALLENGE

90 DAYS TO YOUR PERSONAL BEST

Created By

Combat Veteran John H Davis
NFL Veteran Pat Angerer

#FREEDOMCHALLENGE

TABLE
OF CONTENTS

- The #FreedomChallenge

- Victor Versus Victim

- Victor Well-Being

- The Starting Line

- Tips For Success

- Welcome To Red Phase

- Week 1

- Week 2

- Week 3

- Week 4

- Red Phase Honor Workout

- Red Phase Reflection

- Welcome To White Phase

- Week 5

- Week 6

- Week 7

- Week 8

- White Phase Honor Workout

- White Phase Reflection

- Welcome to Blue Phase

- Week 9

- Week 10

- Week 11

- Week 12

- Blue Phase Honor Workout

- Blue Phase Reflection

- Bonus Ab Workout

- Mission Accomplished

- Our Charity Mission

- Thank You

- About Our Contributors

THE #FREEDOMCHALLENGE

> "How long are you going to wait before you demand the best
>
> for yourself?"
>
> -Epictetus

Self-growth is mandatory in the military and athletic worlds, there's no opting out and declining isn't an option. Each year of service or competition requires a stronger and smarter version of you. You're coached, mentored and there's professional development to encourage you to be your best mental and physical self. Getting out of the military or stopping competing separates you from the built-in challenges those worlds provide. Veterans and athletes need challenges, that's the type of people we are. *The struggles and adversity we face in our lives aren't what make life difficult, they're what make our lives worth living because a challenging life is a purposeful life.*

The #FreedomChallenge is about demanding more from yourself and regaining your edge. It's easy after our past challenges to let that inner fire die out and settle into cruise control within a more comfortable life. But if growth is the goal, then comfort becomes the enemy. Instead of viewing pain and discomfort as the stimulus for growth, we've attempted to eliminate it from our lives. It's time we re-introduce ourselves to the benefits of challenges and beauty of discomfort. *This is the day to be better than who you were yesterday and in 90 days to be the best you that has ever existed.*

Veterans forged this country through blood, sweat, and tears. The greatest moments in American history were Veterans and everyday people facing the toughest of times with courage and conviction. Servicemembers are exposed to a level of hardship most people will never encounter. Veterans have pushed past their limits and faced the unknown in the worst of conditions. Every Veteran has been hungry, dehydrated and sleep deprived. That adversity in the military brings out the best in the men and women that serve. The military forges a team and unites them in a common vision. *Veterans don't run away from a fight, they run to it - this challenge embodies that warrior spirit.*

Athletes are competitors, the driving force is to win. There are early morning practices, difficult training, and a desire for constant improvement. We're not only drawn to sports because of the trophies-we're drawn for the chance to test ourselves. We crave discipline and the pursuit of clear goals. We love how sports brings people together, gives us something to cheer for, and the raw energy of competition.

Athletes are teammates, striving together for victory. An athlete's identity is tied into their sport and stopping competing can remove them from not only their sport, but from themselves. *Success in the athletic world never comes if pain and failure are avoided.*

Whether you're a Veteran, athlete or just someone seeking growth-this is your opportunity to forge new purpose and step firmly into the arena. Taking off the uniform means we lose the growth that service and competition provide. We leave behind that kick in the ass to get up early, push ourselves, and learn new things. Our lives fall into a routine with less stress, obstacles and opponents. There's nothing to train for, no upcoming deployment, and no big game so you're free to hit the snooze alarm. When we lose our team, we also lose the responsibility of being a teammate. *We leave behind a higher purpose and the #FreedomChallenge fills that void.*

Peace has proven itself to be more dangerous for American Veterans than war, we kill ourselves more than the enemy kills us. It's not only the stress that's dangerous for Veterans and civilians alike, but also the lack of positive stress. The mental health epidemic in America affects everyone. Challenges build resiliency, comfort breeds complacency. *The absence of risk is as dangerous as risk because without an enemy to fight, it's easy to go to war with yourself.*

When you rise to meet a challenge, it changes you. We've all been through the highs and lows of life, there's no easy path to victory. Life isn't supposed to be easy and isn't meant to be fair. There's always more to be done. There should never be a point in your life, no matter who you are where you just sit back and say, "that's enough." *You're still in competition against you, that person has always been your biggest opponent... and everything else is only practice.*

There's a difference between working hard and competing*. Other people can force you to work hard but competing comes from within. Everyone that competes works hard but not everyone that works hard competes. We're used to competing with other people throughout our lives, from the school playground to corporate boardrooms. Michael Jordan said, "some people want it to happen, some wish it would happen, others make it happen." By picking up this challenge you're making it happen. *You're always one step away from conquering your life and today you're taking that step.*

....

*Check out Duke's women's basketball coach Kara Lawson's short YouTube video: Working Hard vs. Competing for inspiration

VICTOR VERSUS VICTIM

This challenge will inspire and reawaken your inner warrior to form lifelong victor habits. Life is a series of battles and even if you lose a few, you can still come back and win the war.

There are two spectrums of people. Victors and victims. Picture a coin, on one side is the Archangel Michael, the patron saint of soldiers standing tall and proud. On the other side there is Atlas, condemned to bear the weight of the world on his shoulders, hunched over and beaten down. Michael represents the victors, who pursue challenges, work for opportunities, and assume ownership of their lives. Atlas represents the victims, who have a self-defeating mindset, avoid responsibilities, and fall short of their potential.

The military and sporting worlds have a framework, a set of principles to live by. We trusted ourselves to operate within that system, there was structure that pushed us to be better. The military is organized, athletics are organized, but getting out of the military or stopping competing means that roadmap for success disappears. Envision Neo in the Matrix, he can take the red pill and face reality or the blue pill and stay in a comfortable fantasy. The red pill is the life-changing truth, its freedom accompanied by personal responsibility. It's harder to swallow and uncomfortable. The blue pill goes down smoother. It's an easier road with less obstacles, less responsibility, and you're free to make excuses. This challenge is choosing the red pill and believing the best is yet to come.

Every day is a is a decision of what kind of person to be. The victor mindset is how you win the inner and outer battles we all face. Victors focus on the challenges ahead of them, not the problems of the past. Victors stay on offense in their lives, strive to adopt a growth mindset, and take ownership of their lives. Victors are a force for good, for themselves, their families and their communities. Veterans learn in the military that losing can equal death, but there's also the slow death of a purposeless life.

Nobody consciously chooses to be a victim, but the trap is easy to fall into. We know because we've done it. Discarding the victim outlook means abandoning the widespread "poor me" mentality that's dragging society down. Excuses become a shelter in victimhood, offering protection from the cold truth. The victim mindset is a self-sabotaging, losing mentality that will take over your life if you let it. You defeat it by embracing responsibility for your thoughts, feelings, and actions. Taking on the #FreedomChallenge is swallowing the red pill and the direct path to an unstoppable you. As a victor, you can't own a white flag. There's no surrendering because winning is the only option.

VICTOR WELL-BEING

This challenge isn't a happiness guide or 90 days to a perfect life. Your life needs to get harder before it gets better. There aren't any shortcuts to what we're working towards. It's a difficult journey to develop your full potential and takes zeroing in on your Victor Well-Being. Inside you'll find the tools to navigate your individual path to the best version of yourself. Victor Well-Being has seven specific categories. The #FreedomChallenge works through all of them to create balanced and sustainable growth to carry into your future.

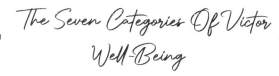

The Seven Categories Of Victor Well-Being

1. Transitional Well-Being: How properly are you adjusted into your post Veteran, post education, or post athletic life? How effectively have you adapted to and handled life's inevitable changes?

2. Physical Well-Being: How healthy is your body? Do you eat right, exercise and get enough sleep? Are you managing, healing, and working through your injuries?

3. Mental Well-Being: How mentally strong do you feel? What attitude are you taking into your day-to-day life? Do you have a Victor mindset?

4. Tribal Well-Being: Are you a member of a community that you contribute to, do you add value to those around you? Do they add value to you?

5. Financial Well-Being: How healthy are you economically? Can you afford all the things you need and some of what you want? Are you economically stressed?

6. Elemental Well-Being: Do you have purpose in your life? Have you discovered your element and how to live it? Do you have something to aim at?

7. Spiritual Well-Being: Do you have a connection with something greater than yourself? How do you deal with the unknown and does your life hold deeper meaning?

THE STARTING LINE

The #FreedomChallenge is split into three 30-day phases: Red, White, and Blue. Each of these phases has different reading, self-growth, and watching recommendations. Each week has workout suggestions submitted by Veterans and athletes. Each week has a specific challenge and discomfort idea to undertake, and each phase is designed to spark balanced growth. All three phases have an honor workout to remember and honor a fallen servicemember. Some of the workouts might go beyond your current fitness levels or capabilities, modify them as needed or choose to do something else. The important thing is your growth, not how you do it.

Potential is a tricky thing, none of us will make all the right life decisions, work as hard as we should, or get as lucky as we want. Personal growth is intentional in the military and athletic worlds, there's a linear path of progression to follow. The modern world is a jungle, but it's best we prepare ourselves for the jungle rather than asking it to change its nature. This challenge is your machete, to cut through that jungle to the other side.

If you've been in the military or been a serious athlete, you've probably had enough of other people telling you what to do. Now it's time for you to tell yourself what to do, and just as importantly – stop doing. Because what we should stop doing is as important as what we should start. All the support in the world doesn't change the reality that personal responsibility and your victor mindset are crucial to your success. This challenge calls out to the warrior in you, to pursue obstacles and fight hard for your future.

Be open to taking on new discomforts, unique experiences, and exploring different types of learning. But you don't have a chain of command or coach in this so if something doesn't fit your needs, then choose something else. The #FreedomChallenge isn't a weight loss-journey, a spiritual quest, or a homework assignment. You'll get out of it what you put into it. If you need a rest day here and there, then take them.

Commit yourself to being a better person in 90 days, there's nothing in these pages beyond your capabilities. There's a lot in here, it's meant to test you. Don't feel like you have to do everything, every day because that's not how growth works. Pain and discomfort are a high cost to pay, but it's the cost of success. Taking on the #FreedomChallenge is paying that price. We're asking you to work as hard for yourself as you do for others over the next 90 days.

TIPS FOR SUCCESS IN ALL THREE PHASES

1. Own the morning. Start your challenge early because if you win the morning, you'll win the day.

2. Enlist allies. Do the challenge with someone to hold each other accountable, find a partner and motivate one another to be your best selves.

3. Cross the days out. Physically X the days out after you complete them, it'll give you a sense of accomplishment. Each day completed builds momentum.

4. Don't throw the towel in. If you miss a day, that happens. The world is going to be hard enough on you, you don't need to be overly hard on yourself.

5. Visualize. Imagine where you want to be in 90 days and then act. See it before you do it.

6. Strategize beforehand. Go into each day with a plan, that's how you'll get ahead. Create structure for yourself and stay organized.

7. Be committed. You're not a bystander in this challenge, you're the star. This is a 90-day growth contract between you and you.

8. Learn on the journey. Highlight in the books, talk to people about the self-growth content to get the most out of the learning experience and reflections.

9. Have some fun. Keep a positive attitude, even through the discomforts. Enjoy the process and remember progress is the best motivator.

10. Eliminate distractions. Lots of things will get in your way if you let them. It's become far too easy to be sidetracked in the modern world.

11. Take an off day. If you feel burned out, take a day off when you need it.

12. Say no. Then say no again to the things that hold you back and prevent your growth. The world will steal your time, money, and future from you if you let it.

13. Keep a routine. The military and sports ingrain solid habits. You get up early, you work hard and you show up day after day. There's great power in daily routines.

14. **Don't neglect your mental health.** Don't take on too much but you aren't a weak candle so easily burnt out. You're stronger than you think. Prioritize your mental, emotional, and spiritual health.

15. **Believe in yourself.** Don't make excuses and don't let people make excuses for you. When you believe in yourself, others will believe in you too.

Tips to Myself

WELCOME TO RED PHASE

Red Phase Rules

1. Stretch each morning
2. Engage with at least 20 minutes of self-growth content per day
3. Exercise twice each day
4. Follow a diet and limit your alcohol
5. Read a chapter each day

. _____

. _____ *

I'm going to stop _____

Examples: Procrastinating, Fast-Food, Staying Up Late, Losing My Temper, etc.

1. It doesn't matter how you stretch, just spend 5 or so minutes before you leave the house stretching out. YouTube has great stretching routines. Warm your body up before attacking the day.

2. There's lots of positive self-growth content out there. Check out the recommendations or choose your own.

3. Two-a-days might seem like too much. It's not. Go jog in the morning and play with your kids at night. Hit the gym in the morning and walk your dog in the afternoon. Whatever floats your boat, just do it twice. Look up a 10-minute YouTube routine for one of your workouts or knock out some push-ups and sit-ups during Netflix.

4. Pay attention to what you eat and cut your alcohol consumption.

5. One chapter, at least, each day. Listen to an audiobook if that's better for you.

....

* Extra space in case to add your own rules if desired, you can add but you can't take away.

RED PHASE RECOMMENDATIONS

Reading

Make Your Bed by William H. McRaven

The Mamba Mentality by Kobe Bryant

Atomic Habits by James Clear

Self-Growth Content

Ted Talk: *How Great Leaders Inspire Action* by Simon Sinek

Podcast: Jocko Podcast #115- *Into the Fire, and Beyond the Call of Duty* with Medal of Honor Recipient Dakota Meyer

Youtube Video: *Get Back Up* by Nick Vujicic

*Watching**

Free Solo directed by Jeremy Chin and Elizabeth Chai Vasarhelyi

Lionness directed by Meg McLagan and Daria Sommers

Pumping Iron directed by George Butler and Robert Flore

....

* Over the course of the month, skip the Netflix one night and throw on one of these documentaries or one similar to inspire you.

RED PHASE CALENDAR

X The Days Out When You Complete Them Or Write In There What Helps You

Red Phase Start Date: ───────────────────────────

Red Phase Completion Date: ─────────────────────

Signature: ────────────────────────────

WEEK 1

Write In What Works For You

	Stretch	Self-Growth Content	Exercise		Diet	Book
M						
T						
W						
T						
F						
S						
S						

Weekly Challenge: Look at alltrails.com and find a hiking path near you. It'll list distances, difficulty, and even let you know things like if it's dog friendly.

Weekly Discomfort: Hop in an ice bath. Buy a bag of ice and throw it in your tub or whatever you can climb into. Get cold, shock your body, and reap the benefits.

Weekly Workouts: *"Robo Shoulders"* by Veteran Robert Cox and *"King Back"* by NFL Player Mitch King

WEEK 1 WORKOUTS

These workouts are suggestions, designed to inspire you and are not mandatory.

"Robo Shoulders"

Submitted by Veteran Robert Cox

- Overhead Barbell Press 4x12
- Dumbbell Shrug 4x12
- Side Raises 4x10
- Kettlebell Swings 4x10
- Cable Upright Row 4x10
- Rear-Delt on Pec-Dec 4x8

"King Back"

Submitted by NFL Player Mitch King

- T Bar Rows 4x8-12
- Lat Pulldowns 4x8-12
- Incline Dumbbell Rows 4x8-12
- Barbell Bent Over Rows 4x8-12
- Pull-ups 3x8-12
- Inverted Back Rows 3x max reps

Weekly Reflection

WEEK 2

Write In What Works For You

	Stretch	Self-Growth Content	Exercise		Diet	Book
M						
T						
W						
T						
F						
S						
S						

Weekly Challenge: Set yourself a lights off time and a wake up time and stick to it every day. When we sleep better, we perform better, and our lives are better.

Weekly Discomfort: Repair a relationship of yours, whether it's a friend, family member, or coworker. Have an uncomfortable conversation and apologize if you need to.

Weekly Workouts: *"Texas Ranger"* by Army Ranger Samuel Brooks and *"Big E Leg Day"* by WWE Champion Ettore Ewen

WEEK 2 WORKOUTS

These workouts are suggestions, designed to inspire you and are not mandatory.

"The Texas Ranger"

Submitted by Army Ranger Samuel Brooks

- A 6-mile ruck march with a bag with 40lbs *
- At the beginning, and every two miles walked and at the end stop to do:
  - 30 Push-ups
  - 30 Second Plank
  - 30 Air Squats
- 10 Minute Stretch At Finish Line

"Big E Leg Day"

Submitted by WWE Champion Ettore Ewen

- Barbell Split Squat 4x5
- Barbell Jumps 4x10
- Front Squats 2x5, 1x4, 2x3
- Cable Pull Throughs 3x15
- Walking Barbell Lunge 3x12
- Seated V-Twist 2x15
- Barbell Complex (Hang Clean, Front Squat, Push Press, Back Squat, Good Morning) 2x6
- Barbell Side Bends 2x10

Weekly Reflection

_____

_____

_____

_____

_____

_____

_____

_____

_____

*If 40 pounds is too much, do 20. If 20 pounds is too much, then just walk. You can do it on a treadmill as well but get outside in nature if possible.

WEEK 3

Write In What Works For You

	Stretch	Self-Growth Content	Exercise	Diet	Book
M					
T					
W					
T					
F					
S					
S					

Weekly Challenge: Do one small thing each day that you've been putting off. Pay the bill, run the errand, organize the space, and do the things you've put on the back burner.

Weekly Discomfort: Find a sauna and sweat it out. Hitting the sauna has a lot of health benefits including detoxification, heart health, stress relief and it just feels good.

Weekly Workouts: *"Take The Bull By The Horns"* by Veteran Dan Colello and *"Strong Island"* by Golden Gloves Champion Kristian Vasquez

WEEK 3 WORKOUTS

These workouts are suggestions, designed to inspire you and are not mandatory.

"Take The Bull By The Horns"

Submitted by Veteran Dan "Bull" Colello

- Pulldown Superset With Triceps Pressdown 4x12
- Dumbbell Row Superset With Dumbbell Kickbacks 4x12
- Cable Row 3x15
- Dumbbell Overhead Extensions 3x15
- Back Extensions 3x12
- Straight Arm Pulldowns 3x12
- Bench Dips Till Failure x3

"Strong Island"

Submitted by boxer Kristian Vasquez

- 3 Rounds Jumprope (3-Minute Rounds 1 Min Rest)
- 4 Rounds Shadow Boxing (3-Minute Round 1 Min Rest)
- Stretch 8-10 Minutes
- 6 Rounds Heavy Bag (3-Minute Round 1 Min Rest)
- 4 Rounds of 25 Push-ups To 30 Crunches
- 25 Minutes Cardio Your Choice

Weekly Reflection

_____

_____

_____

_____

_____

_____

_____

_____

_____

_____

_____

_____

WEEK 4

Write In What Works For You

	Stretch	Self-Growth Content	Exercise		Diet	Book
M						
T						
W						
T						
F						
S						
S						

Weekly Challenge: Use a step counter on your phone, download an app or get a device. Hit 70,000 steps this week. For an extra challenge go 100,000.

Weekly Discomfort: An act of kindness, every day for a week. Pay for a stranger's coffee, give out a compliment every day, and inject some kindness into the world.

Weekly Workouts: *"Dime Piece"* by Veteran Zac Stoltenberg and *"No Defeat"* by athlete Shannon Burge

WEEK 4 WORKOUTS

These workouts are suggestions, designed to inspire you and are not mandatory.

"Dime Piece"

Submitted by Veteran Zac Stoltenberg

- 5x10 Leg extensions
- 5x10 Leg curls
- 5x10 Leg Press
- 5x10 Squat
- 10 Minutes on the stair master
- 5-10 Minute Stretch

"No Defeat"

Submitted by athlete Shannon Burge

- Standing Shoulder Press 50 reps with 3 or 5lb
- Side Raise 50 reps with 3 or 5lb
- Seated Dumbbell Shoulder Press 4x12
- Victory Press 5x15,12,12,15,20
- Side Raise Superset With Low Heavy Partial Side Raise 4x12-15
- High Partial Side Raise 3x30 With 3 or 5lb
- Incline Rear Delt Fly 3x20

Weekly Reflection

_____
_____
_____
_____
_____
_____
_____
_____
_____
_____
_____
_____
_____
_____

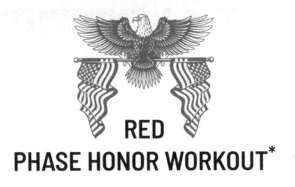

RED
PHASE HONOR WORKOUT*

Red Phase Honor Workout is dedicated to Sean Cutsforth who was KIA Dec 15, 2010 in Afghanistan. He was assigned to 3rd Battalion, 187th Infantry Regiment, 3rd Brigade Combat Team, 101st Airborne Division (Air Assault), Fort Campbell, Kentucky.

We Remember Sean

- Stationary Bike 3 Miles
- Elliptical 2 Miles
- Rower 1,000 Meters
- 100 Sit-ups And 100 Push-ups
- Quiet Reflection And A Moment Of Silence

* Do the Honor Workout whenever works for you throughout the month and as many times as you want to honor Sean. We recommend doing them at the end of the phase to signify your accomplishment and honor this hero.

RED PHASE REFLECTION

What did I learn from my reading?

_____
_____
_____
_____
_____
_____
_____

What did I gain from my self-growth content?

_____
_____
_____
_____
_____
_____
_____
_____

What impacted me from my challenges and my discomforts?

_____
_____
_____
_____
_____
_____
_____
_____

RED PHASE REFLECTION

What inspired me from my documentary choice?

_____

_____

_____

_____

_____

_____

_____

Ask Yourself...

Did I push myself as hard as I should have physically?

_____

_____

_____

Did my month reflect my life priorities the way it should have?

_____

_____

_____

What am I grateful for?

_____

_____

_____

_____

_____

_____

WELCOME TO WHITE PHASE

White Phase Rules

1. Plan each day on a 3x5 card, a post-it note, dry-erase board, or paper
2. Talk to another veteran, athlete, or positive person every day. Find someone doing the challenge and motivate one another.
3. Work out once a day
4. Follow a diet and limit your alcohol
5. Read at least a chapter each day

. _____
. _____ *

I'm going to stop _____
Examples: Mindless Scrolling, Sugar, Not Getting Enough Sleep, Overthinking, etc.

1. Plan your day out, write down your daily tasks. Do it the night before so you wake up and attack the day with a battle plan in mind.

2. We're stronger together. Talk to another Veteran, athlete, or person who uplifts you each day. Intentionally surround yourself with people that inspire you.

3. Keep working out a part of your daily routine and incorporate things you enjoy. Ride a bike, hit a punching bag, or join a softball league. Get outside as much as possible for your workouts.

4. Pay attention to what you eat and cut your alcohol consumption.

5. One chapter, at least, each day. Listen to an audiobook if that's better for you.

....

* Extra space in case to add your own rules if desired, you can add but you can't take away.

WHITE PHASE RECOMMENDATIONS

Reading

The Way Forward: Master Life's Toughest Battles and Create Your Lasting Legacy by Dakota Meyer

The Art of Happiness by the Dalai Lamai and Howard Cutler

Unbroken: A World War II Story of Survival, Resilience, and Redemption by Laura Hillenbrand

Self-Growth Content

Ted Talk: Grit: *The Power Of Passion And Perseverance* by Angela Lee Duckworth

Podcast: Jocko Podcast #221- *The Unimaginable Path of Jonny Kim.* Navy SEAL Combat Medic, Doctor, And Astronaut

Youtube Video: *2011 University of Pennsylvania Commencement Speech* by Denzel Washington

Watching*

Murph: The Protector directed by Scott Mactavish

Tyson directed by James Toback

Murderball directed by Dana Adam Shapiro and Henry-Alex Rubin

* Over the course of the month, skip the Netflix one night and throw on one of these documentaries or one similar to inspire you.

WHITE PHASE CALENDAR

X The Days Out When You Complete Them Or Write In There What Helps You

White Phase Start Date: _____

White Phase Completion Date: _____

Signature: _____

WEEK 5

Write In What Works For You

	Stretch	Self-Growth Content	Exercise		Diet	Book
M						
T						
W						
T						
F						
S						
S						

Weekly Challenge: Look for a race, some type of 5k, half marathon, or obstacle course race in your area and sign up. Do an online challenge if that's what works for you. Find yourself a specific challenge, even if it's months away. Once you commit, you've taken the first step.

Weekly Discomfort: Social media detox. Go for deleting at least one app this week and the more you can detox the better. Twitter, FB, IG, TikTok, Snapchat, Pinterest, and the rest will be there when you get back.

Weekly Workouts: *"The Karate Kid"* by Veteran Bryan Flores and *"Gold Medal Workout"* by Paralympian Andy Yohe

WEEK 5 WORKOUTS

These workouts are suggestions, designed to inspire you and are not mandatory.

"The Karate Kid"

Submitted by Veteran Bryan Flores

- Kettlebell Clean, Squat And Press 3x10
- Medicine Ball Push-ups 1 Hand On Ball 3x10 Each Side
- Russian Twist With Medicine Ball 3x10
- Landmine Or Single Arm Dumbbell Shoulder Press 3x10
- Kettlebell Swing 3x10
- Medicine Ball Slam 3x10
- Burpees 3x10

"Gold Medal Workout"

Submitted by Paralympian Gold Medalist Andy Yohe

- Bike Or Run To A Park That Is 15-20 Minutes Away
- Along The Way, Any Hills Encountered You Have to Sprint Up With Maximum Effort
- 10 Minutes Of Your Favorite Stretches
- Three Rounds: Plank 90 Seconds, 20 Push-ups, And 5 Pull Ups From Anything You Can Hang From
- Run/Bike Home
- Stretch For 5 Minutes

Weekly Reflection

_____

_____

_____

_____

_____

_____

_____

_____

_____

_____

WEEK 6

Write In What Works For You

	Stretch	Self-Growth Content	Exercise	Diet	Book
M					
T					
W					
T					
F					
S					
S					

Weekly Challenge: Drink a gallon of water each day this week, fill it in the morning and finish it before you go to sleep. An estimated 75% of Americans are chronically dehydrated.

Weekly Discomfort: Find one thing each day around your house that you don't use, want, or need anymore and at the end of the week donate 7 items to a local charity or a homeless Veteran shelter. Sometimes we don't own our stuff, our stuff owns us.

Weekly Workouts: *"Operation Zulu"* by Veteran Jessie Virga and *"Athlete Development"* by athlete Matt Rokes

WEEK 6 WORKOUTS

These workouts are suggestions, designed to inspire you and are not mandatory.

"Operation Zulu"

Submitted by Veteran Jessie Virga

- Wide Leg Press 6x15,15.10,10,10,8
- Barbell Back Squat 4x15,10,8,6
- Leg Curl Single Leg 3x12
- Calf Raises 5x20
- Glute Kick Backs 4x15,12,12,8
- Bulgarian Split Squat 3x12
- Bodyweight Hip Extensions 4x12

"Athlete Development"

Submitted by by athlete Matt Rokes

- Every Minute On The Minute (EMOM):
  For 20 Minutes
- 10 Push-ups/5 Pull-ups
- Incline Treadmill:
  Start 4mph/8% Incline
  Complete For 8 Minutes Increasing Incline
  by 1% Each Minute

Weekly Reflection

_____

_____

_____

_____

_____

_____

_____

_____

_____

_____

_____

_____

_____

_____

_____

WEEK 7

Write In What Works For You

	Stretch	Self-Growth Content	Exercise	Diet	Book
M					
T					
W					
T					
F					
S					
S					

Weekly Challenge: Call one person on the phone each day and thank them for something they've done for you. Show gratitude in real ways, especially in ways you've put off from your past or youth.

Weekly Discomfort: The "one more" week. Do one more of everything... one more rep, one more sales call, one more hour studying, one more task completed. Go the extra mile in everything you do this week.

Weekly Workouts: *"Swing For The Fences"* by Veteran Peter Swing and *"All-Star"* by Soccer Player Talla Cisse

WEEK 7 WORKOUTS

These workouts are suggestions, designed to inspire you and are not mandatory.

"Swing For The Fences"

Submitted by Veteran Peter J. Swing

- Mountain Climbers (Four Count) x30
- Crunches x30
- Push-ups x30
- Jumping Jacks (Four Count) x30
- Squats x30
- Leg Lifts x30
- Repeat If Desired

"All-Star"

Submitted by athlete Talla Cisse

- Squats 3x10
- High Knees 3x30 seconds
- Hex Bar Deadlift 3x10
- High Knees 3x30 seconds
- Calf Raises 3x15
- Leg Curl 3x10
- Lunges 3x10
- Russian Twists 3x30 seconds

Weekly Reflection

_____

_____

_____

_____

_____

_____

_____

_____

_____

_____

_____

_____

WEEK 8

Write In What Works For You

	Stretch	Self-Growth Content	Exercise	Diet	Book
M					
T					
W					
T					
F					
S					
S					

Weekly Challenge: Find something physical to do outside of your norm. Take a hot yoga class at a local studio, go to a spin class, or head to a boxing gym.

Weekly Discomfort: Cut someone out of your life that you know you should. No mercy.

Weekly Workouts: *"Firepower"* by Veteran Eric D'arce and *"Buff Body"* by athlete Harold Burge

WEEK 8 WORKOUTS

These workouts are suggestions, designed to inspire you and are not mandatory.

"Firepower"

Submitted by Veteran Eric D'arce

- Machine Chest Flye 12,10,8
- Push Ups 10,10,10
- Lat Pulldown 12,10,8
- Reverse Grip Lat Pulldown 12,10,8
- Incline Barbell Press 12,10,8
- Dumbbell Incline Flye 12,10,8
- Seated Close Grip Rows 12,10,8
- Bent Over Dumbbell Rows 12,10,8

"Buff Body"

Submitted by athlete Harold Burge

- Leg Extensions 4x30,10,10,8
- Lying Leg Curls 4x30,10,10,8
- Barbell Back Squat Superset With 20 Jump Squats 3x10
- Plyo Work in B-Ball Gym Or Long Space
- 1 Set Of Each Down And Back
- Lunges, Leap Frogs, Long Stride Lunges

Weekly Reflection

_____
_____
_____
_____
_____
_____
_____
_____
_____
_____
_____
_____
_____
_____
_____

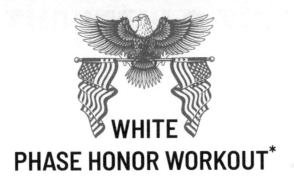

WHITE
PHASE HONOR WORKOUT*

The White Phase Honor workout is dedicated to Staff Sergeant Louis Bonacasa who was killed Dec 21st 2015 in Afghanistan. He was assigned to the 105th Security Forces Sq, Stewart Air National Guard Base, N.Y.

We Remember Louis

- At a local track or on a treadmill
- 400 meter warm up
- Lunge 100 meters, walk 100, lunge 100, walk 100
- 400-meter sprint
- 300-meter sprint
- 200-meter sprint
- 100-meter sprint
- Cool down jog 400 meters

....

* Do the Honor Workout whenever works for you throughout the month and as many times as you want to honor Sean. We recommend doing them at the end of the phase to signify your accomplishment and honor this hero.

WHITE PHASE REFLECTION

What did I learn from my reading and self-growth content?

_____
_____
_____
_____
_____
_____
_____

What did I gain from talking to other veterans and athletes?

_____
_____
_____
_____
_____
_____
_____
_____
_____

What impacted me from my challenges and my discomforts?

_____
_____
_____
_____
_____
_____
_____
_____

WELCOME TO BLUE PHASE

"The truth is you always know the right thing to do.
The tough part is doing it."
-General Norman Schwarzkopf

Blue Phase Rules

1. Get out into nature every day
2. Engage with at least 20 minutes of self-growth content per day
3. Exercise each day
4. Follow a diet and limit your alcohol
5. Read a chapter each day

_____ *

_____

I'm going to stop _____

Examples: Living In The Past, Being Hard On Yourself, Multitasking, Sleeping In, etc.

1. Find yourself in the great outdoors each day. Put your bare feet in the grass, go to a park, or find ways to get outside in whatever ways you can.

2. Check the recommendations or find your own, put it on when you can throughout the day. Make sure you listen to positive content, humor, or self-growth every day.

3. Break a sweat every day. Do it in nature if you want and knock out two birds with one stone. Keep fit and finish this challenge strong.

4. Pay attention to what you eat and cut your alcohol consumption.

5. One chapter, at least, each day. Listen to an audiobook if that's better for you.

* Extra space in case to add your own rules if desired, you can add but you can't take away.

BLUE PHASE RECOMMENDATIONS

Reading

The Art Of War by Sun Tzu

The Book Of Five Rings by Miyamoto Musashi

Man's Search For Meaning by Viktor Frankl

Self-Growth Content

Ted Talk: *What Makes A Good Life?* By Robert Waldinger

Podcast: Jocko Podcast #347: *To Accomplish The Impossible, We Must Decide* With Nick Lavery, Green Beret and Wounded Warrior

YouTube Video: *Choose Your Life – Motivational Speech Compilation* by Motiversity

*Watching**

Alive Day Memories directed by Ellen Goosenberg Kent and Jon Alpert

The Last Dance directed by Michael Tollin

The Barkley Marathon: The Race That Eats Its Young directed by Annika Iltis and Timothy James Kane

....

* Over the course of the month, skip the Netflix one night and throw on one of these documentaries or one similar to inspire you.

BLUE PHASE CALENDAR

X The Days Out When You Complete Them Or Write In There What Helps You

1	2	3	4	5
6	7	8	9	10
11	12	13	14	15
16	17	18	19	20
21	22	23	24	25
26	27	28	30	31

Blue Phase Start Date: _____

Blue Phase Completion Date: _____

Signature: _____

WEEK 9

Write In What Works For You

	Stretch	Self-Growth Content	Exercise	Diet	Book
M					
T					
W					
T					
F					
S					
S					

Weekly Challenge: Give someone one of the books you've finished reading and discuss it with them. This creates your self-growth network.

Weekly Discomfort: Try intermittent fasting, there are a lot of ways to do it. Look up one that works for you.

Weekly Workouts: *"Warpath"* by Veteran Kevin Porter and *"Not Washed Up Yet"* by athlete Tyler Kluver.

WEEK 9 WORKOUTS

These workouts are suggestions, designed to inspire you and are not mandatory.

"Warpath"

Submitted by Veteran Kevin Porter

- Run or Inclined walk 1 mile
- 20 Burpees
- 20 Squats
- 20 Jumping Jacks
- 20 Breaths Plank
- Run or Inclined Walk 2 miles

For Added Intensity Put on a weighted vest or backpack

"Not Washed Up Yet"

Submitted by athlete Tyler Kluver

- 40 Minute ENOM (Every Minute On The Minute)
- Min 1 – 12 Calories Burned on an Air Bike
- Min 2- 12 Toes to Bar
- Min 3- 50 Foot Sled Push
- Min 4- 12 Burpees

Weekly Reflection

_____

_____

_____

_____

_____

_____

_____

_____

_____

_____

_____

_____

WEEK 10

Write In What Works For You

	Stretch	Self-Growth Content	Exercise	Diet	Book
M					
T					
W					
T					
F					
S					
S					

Weekly Challenge: Take a "you" day this week. Clear the fog from your head and do an activity that you love or do nothing at all. Prioritize your wants, needs, and mental health.

Weekly Discomfort: Take a cold shower every day this week in the morning. If that seems insane to you, then end each shower with a 30 second cold burst.

Weekly Workouts: *"Shark Attack"* by Veteran Brian Valero and *"Rock The Morning"* by wrestler Ryan Morningstar.

WEEK 10 WORKOUTS

These workouts are suggestions, designed to inspire you and are not mandatory.

"Shark Attack"

Submitted by Veteran Brian Valero

- Warm Up 5-minute Slow Swim
- 4 Laps Freestyle
- 2 Laps Backstroke
- 2 Laps Freestyle
- 1 Lap Backstroke
- 1 Minute Tread Water With Arms Over Your Head

"Rock The Morning"

Submitted by wrestler Ryan Morningstar

- 10 Minutes Treadmill: Walking On Incline Or Jogging
- Incline Bench Dumbbell Hammer Press (Palms Facing Inward) 5x10
- Seated Kettlebell Or Dumbbell Curl To Press 3x10
- 4x25 Push-ups
- 4x25 Sit-ups
- 100-200 Reps Jump Rope Or Jumping Jacks
- 10-15 Sauna

Weekly Reflection

_____

_____

_____

_____

_____

_____

_____

_____

_____

_____

WEEK 11

Write In What Works For You

	Stretch	Self-Growth Content	Exercise	Diet	Book
M					
T					
W					
T					
F					
S					
S					

Weekly Challenge: : Keep a food journal this week, write down what you're consuming.

Weekly Discomfort: Give something up all week: videogames, caffeine, alcohol, sugar, porn, tobacco, or whatever else. Whatever would create some discomfort and would be good to take a break from.

Weekly Workouts: *"Blind Ninja"* by Veteran Adriel Fernandez and *"Dance Like Nobody's Watching"* by Sai Somboon

WEEK 11 WORKOUTS

These workouts are suggestions, designed to inspire you and are not mandatory.

"Blind Ninja"

Submitted by Veteran Adriel Fernandez

- Mountain Climbers (Four Count) x30
- Crunches x30
- Push-ups x30
- Jumping Jacks (Four Count) x30
- Squats x30
- Leg Lifts x30
- Repeat If Desired

"Dance Like Nobody's Watching"

Submitted by Sai Somboon

- Warmup: 40 Jumping Jacks, 40 Mountain Climbers
- Weighted Lunges 4x10
- Shoulder Press 3x15
- Cardio: 40 Burpees, 40 Knee Raises
- Shoulder Raises 3x15
- Goblet Squat 4x10
- Cardio: 40 Jump Squats, 40 Explosive Push-ups
- Kettlebell Swings 3x15
- Dumbbell Squat Thrusts 3x15

Weekly Reflection

_____

_____

_____

_____

_____

_____

_____

_____

_____

WEEK 12

Write In What Works For You

	Stretch	Self-Growth Content	Exercise	Diet	Book
M					
T					
W					
T					
F					
S					
S					

Weekly Challenge: Spend some time by yourself. Solitude increases productivity, stimulates creativity, and helps you get a better understanding of yourself. Create space to be alone this week.

Weekly Discomfort: Ask three people you trust and respect what you could be doing better and incorporate their constructive criticism into your mindset and life.

Weekly Workouts: *"The Traveler" by Veteran Ron Hurtado and "Bulldog Strength" by athlete Kevin Freking*

WEEK 12 WORKOUTS

These workouts are suggestions, designed to inspire you and are not mandatory.

"The Traveler"

Submitted by Veteran Ron Hurtado

- Shoulder Press 4x12
- Triceps Pressdown 4x10
- Front Raises 4x12
- Skullcrushers 4x10
- Dumbbell Shrug 3x15
- Pec Dec Reverse Flye 3x15
- Dips 3xfailure

"Bulldog Strength"

Submitted by athlete Kevin Freking

- Bench Press Pyramid
- 3x10/3x5/3x1/3x5/3x10
- Dumbbell Flyes 3x10
- Pull-ups 6x5
- Chin-ups 3x5
- 10 Min Treadmill Walk With Incline 12 And Speed 4

Weekly Reflection

_____
_____
_____
_____
_____
_____
_____
_____
_____
_____
_____
_____
_____
_____
_____

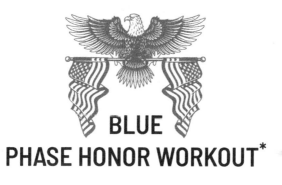

BLUE
PHASE HONOR WORKOUT*

The Blue Phase Honor workout is dedicated to the thirteen servicemembers killed on August 26, 2021, at the Abbey gate during the pullout from Afghanistan.

- Lance Cpl. David Espinoza, 20, of Laredo, Texas
- Sgt. Nicole Gee, 23, of Roseville
- Sgt. Darin Taylor Hoover, 31, of Midvale, Utah
- Army Staff Sgt. Ryan Knauss, 23, of Knoxville, Tenn.
- Cpl. Hunter Lopez, 22, of Indio
- Lance Cpl. Rylee McCollum, 20, of Bondurant, Wyo.
- Lance Cpl. Dylan Merola, 20, of Rancho Cucamonga
- Lance Cpl. Kareem Nikoui, 20, of Norco
- Cpl. Daegan Page, 23, of Omaha, Neb.
- Sgt. Johanny Rosario Pichardo, 25, of Lawrence, Mass.
- Cpl. Humberto Sanchez, 22, of Logansport, Ind.
- Lance Cpl. Jared Schmitz, 20, of Wentzville, Mo.
- Navy Corpsman Maxton Soviak, 22, of Berlin Heights, Ohio

We Remember The 13

To honor the 13 put in thirteen miles

Pick any option

- Ruck 13 miles
- Do a trail walk of 13 miles
- Run 13 miles

Quiet Reflection And A Moment Of Silence

....

* Do the Honor Workout whenever works for you throughout the month and as many times as you want to honor Sean. We recommend doing them at the end of the phase to signify your accomplishment and honor this hero.

BLUE PHASE REFLECTION

What did it feel like making nature a priority?

_____
_____
_____
_____
_____
_____
_____

What ideas did I get from listening to the recommended self-growth content?

_____
_____
_____
_____
_____
_____
_____
_____

What impacted me from my challenges and my discomforts?

_____
_____
_____
_____
_____
_____
_____
_____

BLUE PHASE REFLECTION

What inspired me from my documentary choice?

_____

_____

_____

_____

_____

_____

_____

Ask Yourself...

What do I want people to say at my funeral?

_____

_____

_____

_____

Who around me is influencing my life negatively?

_____

_____

_____

_____

What's really important going forward and as importantly, what's not?

_____

_____

_____

_____

_____

_____

⊩⊢ BONUS AB WORKOUT ⊣⊩

This Ab workout was created by Drill Sergeant and Fitness Competitor Christina Christiansen, a Mother, Soldier, and Athlete.
Christina can be contacted at @christinachristiansen10 on IG

Climb The Ladder Challenge

1. Lay in the supine position and place your hands with fingers interlocked behind your head. Begin doing **crunches** with your legs flat on the ground. Remember to squeeze your core and do them slowly. **Complete 25 Reps**

2. While keeping your back on the ground, bring your knees up and keep your feet flat on the ground. **Complete 25 crunches.**

3. Cross your right leg over your left knee. Bring your left elbow to your right knee. **Complete 25 Reps**

4. Switch your left knee over your right knee. Bring your right elbow to your left knee. **Complete 25 Reps**

5. Bring your right leg straight up in the air. Cross your left leg over the right knee. Bring your right elbow towards your left knee. **Complete 25 Reps**

6. Switch and bring the left straight up in the air with your right leg over the left knee. Bring the left elbow towards the right knee. **Complete 25 Reps.**

7. Bring both legs straight up in the air. **Complete 25 crunches** towards your feet.

Step 7 is the top of the ladder.... What goes up must come down! In reverse order, go down the ladder by doing steps 6 – 1 to complete the challenge.

MISSION ACCOMPLISHED

Congratulations!

Now what? Hell, we don't know. But you're in a better position than when you started. Nobody ever said the journey to be the best version of yourself was supposed to be easy. We chose to walk this difficult path and there's no turning back. Once you serve, you're a veteran for life. Once you compete, you're forever an athlete. Once you've completed the **#FreedomChallenge**-you're a warrior.

We've known too many Veterans, athletes, and people who have done incredible things and then slowly lose their challenges, competitive spirit and even themselves. The victim mentality is too easy of a trap in today's technology world to fall into. Being a victim means you don't have to accept responsibility and you aren't concerned about failing because you won't even try. We've seen society become more individualized, but life isn't supposed to be a solo mission, it's a team game. Community is vital to victor well-being, and we'd like to welcome you to the #FreedomChallenge community. Completing this challenge means you've bettered yourself and you should be proud of that. Throughout our lives we spend a lot of time rooting for other people and cheering their successes while downplaying our own accomplishments. Celebrate your growth, pop some champagne and acknowledge that you're in a better place now than you were 90 days ago.

The end of anything is also the beginning of something else. Your self-growth doesn't belong contained within the pages of this journal, continue it into your future. Spread the Victor Mindset. We're supposed to grow and change throughout our lives, reaching our potential means evolving. We've come to think of pain as something we should avoid and comfort as something we should seek but the opposite is true. For victors to live a life to be proud of, it means getting some bumps and bruises along the way because scars equal stories. It's vital to have a mission to accomplish, mountains to climb and obstacles to overcome. To say hello to the new you, sometimes it takes saying farewell to the old version. Experiencing new things means saying goodbye to some of the old things.

If you failed at this challenge, then shake it off and try again. We've both failed a lot too. But as victors, as athletes and Veterans we have to keep fighting the good fight. Nobody makes it through life without physical, emotional, or mental pain. No one is immune from the stress, trauma, sickness, or addictions life throws at us. We might not win every battle, but victors always win the war. The word victor has a Latin root of vict which means to conquer, and there's still a lot of conquering left to do.

When we leave victimhood, we aren't only escaping from something but also to something. A brighter future when we accept responsibility and seek progress. This challenge forged a path for you and it's your mission to stay on it. Even people who are high performers can fall into complacency if they aren't occasionally tested and pushed to challenge themselves.

Veterans signed up, raised their right hands and were willing to die for our freedoms. Servicemembers have given humanitarian aid, responded to disasters, fought against diseases, and helped people all over the world. People respect veterans. That respect should be used to be voices of common sense, community, and promoting military values. Veterans have done a lot for this country and the country should do more for them.

Military Values

Army Values: *Loyalty, Duty, Respect, Selfless Service, Honor, Integrity, And Personal Courage*
Air Force Values: *Integrity First, Service Before Self, And Excellence In All We Do*
Navy and Marine Values: *Honor, Courage, And Commitment*
Coast Guard Values: *Honor, Respect, and Devotion To Duty*
Space Force Values: *Organizational Agility, Innovation, And Boldness*

On John's website there are articles, books, and other resources. What matters going forward is that we keep challenges a part of our lives no matter who or where we are. We need to keep training, reading and learning. Be a victor and be a winner because your family needs you to be. If you liked the challenge, do it again or share it with someone else. Let us know what you got out of the challenge and use the tag **#FreedomChallenge** on social media. Take a minute to review the challenge on Amazon and more importantly, keep working to spread the Victor mindset.

If you're interested in submitting a workout, discomfort, or challenge to the **#FreedomChallenge2.0**, email John. If you have a fallen veteran or first responder that you'd like to honor for the next challenge, please send us their information and story as well.

Thanks,

John and Pat

OUR CHARITY MISSION

Part of the proceeds from this challenge are donated to the nonprofit organization Suicide Awareness and Remembrance Flag (SAR). Their primary mission is to break the stigma of mental health, suicide and seeking treatment within the warrior culture to facilitate suicide prevention.

We want to thank you for contributing to this important mission with us and to inform you of SAR's goal to get September 22nd annually recognized as "Veteran Suicide Awareness & Remembrance Day" as well as getting the SAR flag congressionally recognized.

There are still 20 veteran and active duty servicemembers that commit suicide every day in this country. That's 7,300 each year, a shocking number. One of the biggest mental health boosters is having purpose and community, we wanted this challenge to provide both. You're now part of the #FreedomChallenge community, where Veterans, athletes and everyone else comes together for the betterment of ourselves, our communities and our country.

If you're interested in learning more about SAR, founded by Veteran Kevin W. Hertell, check out their website at SARFLAG.org or on IG at @SAR_honorthefallen. You can buy the SAR flag to fly, check out merchandise and learn about the importance of their work. We're honored to partner with them to bring attention and resources to Veteran mental health. Thank you, Kevin, to you and your team for all that you do and will continue to do for Veterans, the military community and the country. We are grateful for you.

This challenge isn't just about making you better, it's about giving back, closing the civilian/military gap, and making the world a better place. Thank you for being a part of the #FreedomChallenge family. Look out for the #FreedomChallenge2.0 where we will take on another worthy charity mission, bring forth more challenges, discomforts and get better together.

THANKS

We'd like to thank you for taking this journey with us and getting out of your comfort zone. This challenge came together after our conversations wanting and needing a challenge after Pat retired from the NFL and John from the military. We realize we didn't grow despite the storms and aversities we encountered-we grew because of them. We wanted to provide that for other people based on our combined experiences in the military and athletic worlds.

A person needs hardships to reach their potential like carbon needs pressure and heat to become a diamond. Failure in life is never final, it's a formative event. It's important to fail, feel pain and embrace discomforts on the march to success. Sometimes we win our battles just by having the courage to ride out the storm, to hold on a little longer and survive. We can only figure out how high we can rise when we push our limits. Thank you for pushing yours. We'd like to thank the people that pushed us over the years, from our coaches, leaders, friends, and teammates.

Pat: I'd like to thank my wife Mary, for all her support and selflessness throughout our relationship. My children for giving me a why on days I didn't think I had one. My parents and my siblings for being great role models. The coaches that held me to a higher standard than I held myself. The teammates that fought beside me and my opponents that held me accountable if I wasn't up to par. I'm thankful to be born where I was and surrounded by the people I was. I'm thankful for John and the men and women that have served this country.

John: I'd like to thank my mother for her steadfast belief in me over the years through my personal struggles. My three brothers for showing me brotherhood before I set foot in a combat zone. I'd like to thank my grandfather John Howes. I'd like to thank the people I served with, all over the world who held the line and tried to do the impossible. I'd like to thank the everyday Americans who have made me proud to fight for them. I want to express my heartfelt gratitude for the families of the men and women who have died for America, her ideals, and our freedoms.

We'd like to thank Kevin Freking, Matt Drinkall, Randy Scott, Aaron Wiley, and the Bettendorf Football Staff. We'd also like to thank Norm Parker, Chris Doyle, Kirk Ferentz, Darrel Wilson, Aaron Schwengler, Daniel Wilhite, Nathan Macdougall, and Allen Lynch.

WHO WOULD YOU LIKE TO THANK?

This space is for you to write who you're thankful for, who contributed to your journey, your mindset, or positively impacted you. Either on this challenge or throughout your life.

ABOUT OUR CONTRIBUTORS

We'd like to thank our friends, role models, and heroes for contributing a workout to the
#FreedomChallenge

Robert Cox- Robert is a combat veteran of Iraq and Afghanistan. He's a gamer, tattoo artist, photographer, podcaster, house renovator, and all-around crazy person. Rob lives in Germany with his wife Sylvia and two kids.

Mitch King- Mitch is a 1st Team All American Football Player, 1st Team All-Big Ten, Team Captain of the Iowa Hawkeyes, and played in the NFL for the Tennessee Titans.

Samuel Brooks- Sam is an Army Ranger, Bronze star and Purple heart recipient, and American badass. Sam's somewhere actively serving in the military, protecting our freedoms with his wife Kara and their three kids.

Ettore Ewen- Big E is a WWE Champion, USA Powerlifting Champion, 2X WWE Intercontinental Champion, 6X Smackdown Tag Team Champion, Former NXT Champion, and former NCAA Division 1 Football Player. @wwebige

Dan Colello- Dan is a National Guard Veteran who served in Iraq. Dan is the President of a chapter of the United States Military Vets Motorcycle Club and has received numerous awards for his Veteran advocacy work. He served 25 years of service and continues to train hard, serve his community, and set the standard.

Kristian Vasquez- Kristian is a 2x New York Golden Gloves Champion and owner of @strongislandboxing in New York, Elite Technical Boxing Trainer, Podcaster, and fight promotor. Check him out at www.strongislandboxing.com

Zac Stoltenberg- Zac is an Air Force veteran who served in Afghanistan and throughout the Middle East. He's a sports enthusiast, faith counselor, and adoption advocate. @Zac_Stoltenberg

Shannon Burge- Shannon is a life coach, national fitness competitor, and former NCAA athlete. Check out Shannon's killer workouts, programs, and more at nodefeat.co or @Shannon_Burge on Instagram. Shannon continues to compete, inspire, and serve others.

Bryan Flores- Bryan is a Karate champion and was a member of the USA Karate Senior National Team. He's also a combat Veteran of Iraq and Afghanistan and loves living a full life, coaching, and spending time with his two sons and his wife Tawnie.

Andy Yohe- Andy was team captain of the US Paralympic Ice Sled Hockey team, bringing home the gold medal. Andy lost both of his legs and battled back to become a Paralympian, Gold Medalist, and World Champion.

Jessie Virga- Dr. Jessie Virga is a Navy veteran, CEO of Mulier Bellator Fitness, physique and Brazilian Jiu Jitsu competitor. Check Jessie out at https://www.mbfitnessusa.com/ where she has workouts, mental health resources, and raises money for veteran and first responder causes.

Matt Rokes- Matt is a Doctor of Physical Therapy and co-owner of the Athlete Development Project. He's a collegiate director of Strength and Conditioning. https://www.adpqc.com/

Peter J. Swing- Peter is a Marine and Operation Enduring Freedom Veteran. He is the founder and head of school of Berkeley Academy for Multicultural Studies in Costa Rica. He's a graduate of Harvard and delivers lectures on multiculturalism, history, education, and ethnic studies. He's married to his wife Yorlenny and has three sons.

Talla Cisse- Talla is an avid soccer player and athlete. He works for the United Nations and runs the nonprofit Foundation For A Healthier Senegal providing much needed healthcare, nutrition, and education in rural communities in Africa. Check out Talla's foundation at fohsen.org

Eric D'arce- Eric is Marine Veteran and MMA competitor with a background in Taekwondo. He's a Veteran mental health advocate, father, and a Student Veterans of America Chapter President. Eric is engaged to Jeslie Alvarado and has three children. Eric turned his own mental health struggles into his passion to help other veterans.

Harold Burge- Harold is a life-changing ISSA Multi-Certified Trainer with multiple 1st place finishes winning NPC Men's Physique Competitions. He's a realtor in Iowa on top of being a fitness competitor, role model, and trainer. Harold can be reached through IG at @reignjagger_ and @thebuffcompany

Kevin Porter- Kevin is an Army veteran, Paratrooper and author of *Joining The Military: Everything You Need To Know Your Recruiter Won't Tell You*. Kevin is an entrepreneur and outdoor adventure enthusiast.

Tyler Kluver- Tyler played football at the University of Iowa where he was an All Big Ten specialist, is a fitness and nutrition coach, and is the host of the @washedupwalkons podcast. Check out his programs at www.tylerkluver.com

Brian Valero- Brian is a combat veteran of Afghanistan and veteran advocate. Brian is an active volunteer and organizer for the Veterans of Foreign Wars and The Disabled American Veterans. He's very much in love with his country and his wife, poet Natasha Desiree.

Ryan Morningstar- Ryan is a 2x All-American wrestler and the member of three NCAA Championship teams. Ryan is also a NCAA Championship winning coach, a three-time state champion, and qualified for the US Olympic Team Trials.

Adriel Fernandez- Adriel is a blind Navy Veteran. He continues to inspire and compete, racing in triathlons, training jiu-jitsu, and telling his story to show anything is possible. Adriel is a veteran, competitive athlete, husband, and father. Find Adriel on Youtube or social media: @blindninja.

Sai Somboon- Sai is a theatre director, fitness instructor, professional dancer/actor, and youth mentor. He's the Associate Director of College Counseling at the Dalton School. Sai is also a stand-up comedian in the NYC area. @Sai_the_thai

Ronald Hurtado- Ron is a combat Veteran of Iraq and Afghanistan, founder of the Airborne Tri Team, and volunteers in Latin America to connect kids with sports, competition, and personal betterment.

Kevin Freking- Kevin is a former powerlifter and competitive cyclist. He's a strength and conditioning coach who has impacted thousands of athletes through his training, coaching, and outreach efforts.

Christina Christiansen- Christina is a fitness competitor, mother, and Drill Sergeant who is continuing to serve this country, protect our freedoms, and be a role model.

If you're interested in submitting a workout to be featured in the **#FreedomChallenge2**
then reach out to

john.h.davis.writer@gmail.com
or
@john.h.davis.writer on IG.

Thanks Again to our Contributors!

Made in the USA
Middletown, DE
28 September 2023

39667896R00038